Holy Glow Grail

If You've Ever Googled "Is This Healthy?"—This Book

Is for You

by Margot Reed

"This book wasn't a manual. It was a glow-up group chat in book form. The kind you open during errands, scroll before bed, or shove at your best friend with a 'Read this, it's literally us.'"

Read This First

Margot Reed is a pen name, but the glow is very real.

Behind the alias is a woman with a husband, three boys, a dog, a garden, and more Amazon subscriptions than she's willing to admit. She's a former analyst, small business owner, political campaign staffer, and medical manuscript editor who now reads clinical trials like beach novels and follows functional medicine doctors like most people follow celebrities.

Her wellness journey started after a melanoma diagnosis (she doesn't lead with it, but it lit the match), and became a full-blown obsession with figuring out what works. Spoiler: it's not whatever's trending—it's whatever helps you wake up looking suspiciously like you're still in your twenties, even when you're very much not.

This isn't a book written by a doctor. It's written by a girl who has read 14 studies before electrolytes + coffee and still makes time for squats, school pickup, and a weeknight glass of wine—not to impress you, but to show you that you can too.

You won't find gatekeeping here. No overpriced routines. No shamey advice. No 58-step morning rituals that only work if you have a house manager and a private sauna. Just real, researched, glow-up strategies for real life.

She's lived the chaotic, caffeine-fueled, kid-chasing life—and still found ways to glow from the inside out. Her goal? Show you how to do it, too—without the overwhelm. This book is what your group chat would look like if it came with citations and clear skin. A little rebellious, a little refined, and unfiltered.

Let's glow.

—Margot

Table of Contents

Introduction
Welcome to Glow Mode

This isn't just a summer guide. It's your reset button.

Whether you're 26 or 46, single or juggling three kids and a calendar that never stops, *Glow Mode* is your invitation to return to yourself—and bring your glow.

To glow doesn't just mean you look good. It means you feel grounded, clear, and confident. It's the moment you finally drink water before coffee. It's slicking your hair into a ponytail—not because anyone's watching, but because you want to feel pulled together. It's zinc-based SPF, a cold face towel, and a quiet "I've got this" before the world comes knocking.

Maybe you're new to wellness. Perhaps you've done this before and you're coming back to it—older, wiser, and honestly just too tired for anything that feels complicated or fake. Either way, this book meets you where you are and walks with you forward.

No overhauls. No guilt. Just simple, energizing rituals to support your real life.

Inside, you'll find:

- Real meals made without seed oils (that taste good)

- Micro-workouts that reset your mood in under 15 minutes
- Style and skincare that doesn't cost a fortune or your soul
- Rituals to calm your mind and lift your cheekbones (literally)
- Printable habit trackers, glow badges, and weekly challenges to keep you going

To the moms:

You don't need a full hour. You need two minutes and a reminder that *you matter, too*. While the coffee brews, the baby naps, and the house is half asleep, you can stretch, sip lemon water, or press frozen peas to your cheekbones. That's the work. That's the beginning.

You're not behind. You're ready.

This is for the woman tired of feeling like she's always catching up. It is for the woman who wants to feel powerful in her body again and who misses how fun it felt to care for herself before everything else got louder.

Glow Mode On is about reclaiming your energy, confidence, and joy. It's about making wellness feel personal again. Playful again. *Real* again.

So grab your notebook. Your water. Your face mist—or your bag of frozen peas.

Pull your hair back into a Kris Jenner ponytail facelift.

And let's turn the light back on.

Chapter 1: Glow Starts Here

Hot Girl Habits: Your Daily Glow Foundation

Forget hustle. Forget perfection. *Glow Mode* is about rhythms that support you, not stress you out. These are the real habits of women who glow—even when life is a mess and the kids cry in the next room.

This isn't a complete makeover. It's a reset. Small, consistent rituals that tell your body and brain: "We're safe, we're worthy, and we're choosing energy today."

The Morning Stack (takes 10–15 minutes):

- Drink water with lemon and a pinch of sea salt.
- Look in the mirror and say one kind sentence to yourself. "Today I show up as the version of me I admire."
- Do two minutes: arms overhead, shoulder rolls, and one slow, intentional breath.
- Add a glow moment using what you already have. Splash cold water on your face. Try an ice face bath. Use your moisturizer with slow, upward strokes. If you use SPF, make it zinc-based. That matters.

Eat to Stabilize, Not Shrink

No skipping. No starving. No apologies for needing food. Real nourishment supports your mood, skin, hormones, and energy. That's the glow.

Glow Fuel Basics:

- Eat a full breakfast with protein and healthy fats.
- Avoid seed oils (we'll break this down in Chapter 3).
- A spoonful of coconut oil or ghee mid-morning helps support hormones.
- Keep snacks authentic and satisfying. Try cheese cubes, hard-boiled eggs, olives, or berries.

Walk Like You Mean It

Your body was made to move, and your mind is begging for fresh air and endorphins. A 15-minute walk can reset your mood, reduce inflammation, clear brain fog, and maybe even change your day.

Put on your favorite playlist or your go-to comfort show. Something familiar. Something fun. You know the one. Toss your phone in your Lulu crossbody or plug in some wired headphones—because yes, retro is trending, and no, Bluetooth isn't cute for your nervous system.

Walk tall. Breathe deeper. Let the sun hit your cheekbones. You're not just taking a walk. You're reclaiming your glow, one step at a time.

Goal: Walk four times this week. That's it.

Nighttime Wind Down

Your glow builds while you sleep. Help it along by ending your day with calm and consistency.

Evening Wind-Down Routine:

- Turn off screens at least 30 minutes before bed.
- Stretch while brushing your teeth.
- Use the body lotion you already have and apply it with care.
- Write down one good thing from your day, even if it's "I survived."

No perfection required—just consistency and kindness.

5-Day Hot Girl Habit Challenge

Check off each of the following habits five days in a row. You don't need to do them perfectly. You need to show up.

Progress builds momentum, and momentum builds glow.

Habit	Mon	Tue	Wed	Thu	Fri
Lemon water + stretch					
Mirror affirmation					
Real breakfast (no oils)					
Walk (or movement reset)					

Habit	Mon Tue Wed Thu Fri

Night wind-down

Complete the full grid? You've earned your first Glow Badge.

Weekly Affirmation

"I am 30% water, 70% ambition, and currently held together by zinc sunscreen and delusional confidence."

Chapter 2: Fit Girl Energy

Reset Your Body, Reclaim Your Confidence

Before we begin: stop comparing yourself to Instagram reels. Yes, you do it. We all do. But here's your permission slip to not go there today. That girl's "what I eat in a day" is probably filtered, edited, and eaten under a ring light. This is real life. Your life. And you don't need a trending audio to prove your glow.

"We're not here to chase skinny. We're here to chase energy, strength, and the joy of catching your reflection and thinking, 'Okayyy, who's she?'"

This chapter isn't about losing weight or "fixing" your body. It's about reclaiming it—day by day, rep by rep. The goal is to feel stronger, clearer, and more present in your skin.

You don't need fancy equipment. You don't need a gym. You need a plan, a sense of humor, and maybe two soup cans. That's enough.

We're breaking it down into four settings, so there's no excuse to skip it. Do it at home, outside, in the gym, or in a hotel. Wherever you are, your glow follows.

Let's move.

Home Workouts: The No-Pants Program

Perfect for pajama mornings or post-dinner movement. You can do this barefoot while catching up on your favorite comfort show. Romanticize it. You're in your living room doing lunges while Olivia Pope solves another scandal. Yes, queen.

Quick Home Circuit (12 minutes)

Repeat two rounds:

- 15 bodyweight squats
- 10 countertop pushups
- 20 standing knee lifts (10 each side)
- 30-second wall sit
- 10 tricep dips on a chair
- 30 seconds of dancing or jumping jacks

Glow Tip: Use soup cans, shampoo bottles, or whatever's in your cabinet as weights. Play music you love and pretend you're in a training montage.

Outside Workouts: Romanticize the Walk

Walking is medicine. Don't underestimate it. Walk like it's a scene in your biopic. Skip the shades—catch that morning sun on your face. Carry your phone in your Lululemon crossbody. Turn the volume up. Wear wired headphones if you're feeling vintage.

Outdoor Circuit (15–20 minutes)

- 10-minute walk at any pace

- 15 walking lunges per leg
- 15 standing leg lifts per side
- 1-minute stair step (or curb step-up)
- 5-minute walk home

Glow Tip: Spray perfume just for this. Breathe deep. Call it your "glow lap."

Gym Workouts: No Wandering, Just Winning

You made it to the gym. Let's make it count without wasting time—no scrolling between sets. No overthinking. Just move with purpose and get out of there glowing.

Full-Body Gym Set (20–25 minutes)

Repeat three rounds:

- 12 dumbbell goblet squats
- 10 cable or seated rows
- 12 dumbbell chest presses
- 10 walking lunges per leg
- 5-minute incline treadmill walk (10% incline)

Glow Tip: Wear something that makes you feel good. Hydrate like you mean it. Use the mirror for form, not judgment.

Hotel or Travel Workouts: No Excuses, Just Energy

Hotel gym closed? No problem. You've got 6 feet of floor space and a body that's ready to move.

10-Minute Hotel Circuit

Repeat two rounds:

- 20 air squats
- 10 pushups (knees or full)
- 30-second plank
- 15 glute bridges
- 30-second jog in place

Glow Tip: Open the curtains. Play jazz or lo-fi. Make it feel like a private retreat.

7-Day Glow Movement Challenge

Each day, choose a straightforward move. Commit to doing it. No overthinking. No negotiating. Just press play on your show and move.

Day	Move	Instructions	Glow Cue
Monday	Wall Sit	3 x 30 seconds	Do it during your show's intro
Tuesday	Plank	3 x 20 seconds	Light a candle and breathe through it
Wednesday	Dance Break	3 full songs	Pretend you're in a music video
Thursday	Pushups	3 x 10 (on knees or toes)	Bonus: play a hype anthem

Friday	Stoop Squats	3 x 15 reps	Outside, with coffee or tea
Saturday	Walk + Water	20-minute walk + hydrate	Wear gloss and cute sunglasses
Sunday	Stretch + Breathe	10 minutes of slow flow or yoga	Add soft music and stretch with care

Complete the whole week? You've earned your "Glow in Motion" badge. Bonus points if you feel smug.

Weekly Affirmation

"My glow is lifting cheekbones, moods, and standards—one squat and smug stretch at a time."

Chapter 3: Unfollowed: Canola, Soybean, & Friends

Eat Like You Glow

We're not doing sad salads. We're not skipping meals. We're not counting anything.

We eat to feel clear, energized, and satisfied—and just the right amount. "I eat like I care about myself, *and it shows*" energy. Not because the internet told us to. Because it *feels good*.

You know the drill—you fall down a Reels rabbit hole watching people make homemade sourdough or perfectly prepped mason jar salads for the week. At first, you're inspired and then overwhelmed. And suddenly you're eating crackers over the sink at 8 p.m.

This chapter is the antidote to that. No stress. No batch-cooking marathons. Just authentic meals you can make. You don't need to become someone else. You need a fridge that helps you glow.

This chapter is about building real meals that support your glow from the inside out. That means no seed oils, sugar crashes, or "health" food that leaves you hungry an hour later. Your hormones, skin, and brain will love smart, delicious, glow-up meals.

A Quick Note About Seed Oils

Seed oils sound healthy because marketing told you they were. But most are highly processed, inflammatory, and secretly hiding in everything from oat milk to salad dressing. You don't need to be perfect, but you do need to be aware. And this chapter is your awareness training.

If you take nothing else from this chapter, take this: check the label. If it says canola, soybean, sunflower, safflower, grapeseed, corn, or vegetable oil? That's a no. If it says butter, ghee, *organic* olive oil (look for the harvest date), tallow, coconut oil, or avocado oil? You're golden.

Why I Choose Organic (and Why You Might Want To)

This isn't about being fancy—it's about avoiding chemicals your glow doesn't need. Most non-organic produce in the U.S. is sprayed with glyphosate, a weed killer linked to hormone disruption, gut issues, and chronic inflammation.

Choose organic, especially for foods where you eat the skin (like berries, greens, and apples) when possible. If it's not within the budget, there is no stress. Just wash the produce well and make the best choice you can. You're still doing amazing.

What to Eat More Of

This isn't a diet. It's a reset. Add more of these, and you'll naturally eliminate the junk.

- Organic eggs cooked in butter
- Wild-caught salmon or sardines
- Grass-fed ground beef with real sea salt
- Roasted veggies with ghee or coconut oil
- Full-fat Greek yogurt with berries
- Dark chocolate (yes, seriously)
- Avocados, olives, raw cheese, and nuts (if tolerated)

What to Eat Less Of (But Still Be Chill About It)

We're not demonizing. We're just being real. These foods mess with your energy, skin, mood, and metabolism.

- Seed oils
- Ultra-processed "low-fat" snacks
- Anything that spikes blood sugar and crashes it
- Store-bought sauces, dressings, and protein bars pretending to be healthy
- Coffee before breakfast (eat first, then caffeinate)

Your Glow Kitchen Staples *(organic if possible)*

Here's what to keep in your kitchen for fast, glow-worthy meals:

- Butter, ghee, coconut oil
- Organic eggs, cheese, frozen wild salmon, or grass-fed beef
- Avocados, lemons, frozen berries
- Full-fat Greek yogurt (plain)
- Canned tuna or sardines
- Dark chocolate, raw honey
- Real salt (like Redmond's or sea salt)

Screenshot-Worthy Grocery List

(Save this in your notes or screenshot for your next haul.)

Proteins

- Organic eggs
- Grass-fed ground beef
- Wild-caught salmon or sardines
- Full-fat Greek yogurt (plain)
- Canned tuna (in olive oil)
- Raw cheese
- Grass-fed beef sticks (like Chomps)

Fats & Pantry Staples

- Butter, ghee, coconut oil

- Avocados
- Raw nuts (almonds, walnuts, Brazil nuts)
- Chia seeds
- Raw honey
- Real salt (sea salt or Redmond's)

Produce

- Leafy greens (spinach, arugula)
- Zucchini, onions, carrots
- Lemons and limes
- Frozen berries
- Sweet potatoes

Extras

- Dark chocolate (70%+ cacao)
- Coconut butter packets
- Herbal tea or sparkling water

---

5 Glow Meals You Can Make On Repeat

1. Lemon-Butter Wild-Caught Salmon with Veggies
   Bake salmon with butter, lemon, and salt. Serve with
   steamed broccoli and sweet potato.
2. Egg Bowl with Avocado and Hot Sauce
   Scrambled or fried eggs, avocado slices, salsa, and
   greens. Add cheese if it's that kind of day.

3. Taco Bowl Without the Gut Bomb

   Ground beef, avocado, shredded cheese, and a squeeze of lime. Serve over cauliflower rice or lettuce.

4. Berry Yogurt Bowl

   Full-fat Greek yogurt, frozen blueberries, chia seeds, cinnamon, and a drizzle of raw honey.

5. Roasted Veggies with Ghee and Sea Salt

   Toss carrots, zucchini, and onions in ghee. Roast at 400°F until caramelized. Serve with meat or eggs.

The "Don't Get Hangry" Plan

You're not glowing if you're snapping. Keep one of these on hand at all times:

- Cheese sticks
- Boiled eggs
- Olives
- Grass-fed beef sticks
- Coconut butter packets
- A spoonful of peanut butter (organic & seed oil free!)

Weekly Glow-Up Food Challenge

Try one new glow meal every day this week. Snap a pic. Romanticize the plate. Make it a moment.

Day	Meal	Did it?
Monday	Lemon-Butter Salmon	
Tuesday	Egg Bowl	
Wednesday	Taco Bowl	
Thursday	Yogurt + Berries	
Friday	Roasted Veggie Tray	
Saturday	Anything with Avocado	
Sunday	Your Favorite, Seed-Oil-Free Style	

Weekly Affirmation

"I eat like someone who knows her skin, hormones, and sanity depend on it—because they do."

Chapter 4: Margs, Mindfulness, & Main Character Energy

Glow Through the Weekend

You know how it goes—Friday hits, your group chat is blowing up, and suddenly your "clean girl" week collides with a dirty martini and a plate of truffle fries. And then the next morning? You're deep in someone's "What I Eat in a Day" video, wondering if oat milk is ruining your life and why everyone on TikTok seems to have a perfect morning routine *even after bottomless brunch.*

Pause. Breathe. You didn't ruin anything.

This chapter is your weekend survival kit—with zero shame attached.

Because yes, we're glowing. But we're also going out. We're celebrating. We're ordering dessert sometimes, and not spiraling when the fries were probably fried in soybean oil. It's not about being perfect. It's about being *cognizant*. That's the word of the chapter. Knowing how to support your body even when life gets a little loud.

First Glow Tip: Hydration Is More Than Water

You chug three glasses of water and still feel dry? Yeah, that's because water alone doesn't hydrate you.

Proper hydration needs minerals, especially salt. When you sweat, drink alcohol, or stress-scroll TikTok for 45 minutes straight, your body loses electrolytes. Plain water without salt... flushes more of them out.

That's where electrolytes come in.

Add a pinch of sea salt and a squeeze of lemon to your water, or use a clean electrolyte mix like Re-Lyte. There are no sugar bombs or dyes—just the minerals your glow needs to bounce back.

After a night out, your recovery drink isn't green juice—it's salted water in a cute cup.

If You're Drinking, Read This

You don't have to give up alcohol to feel good, but understanding that your body works harder to detox from it can help you plan.

Here's the hierarchy, listed from least to most inflammatory:

- Top Shelf: Organic tequila or mezcal with soda water and lime

- Next Best: Vodka or gin with fresh citrus

- Avoid If You Can: Sugary mixers, canned cocktails, and bottom-shelf anything
- Red Alert: Beer, flavored seltzers, and sweet wines (hello, sugar and seed oils)

Glow Strategy:

Eat first. Sip slowly. Alternate with water. Add sea salt to your morning after.

Your Non-Alcoholic Power Moves

Not drinking? You're still glowing, and your drink should too. Try one of these:

- Sparkling water with lime and mint (in a wine glass)
- Mock margarita: Lime, splash of orange juice, salt rim
- Coconut water + splash of pineapple
- Bitters + soda for a grown-up, not-too-sweet vibe

Make it look cute. Feel included—no hangover.

What to Eat Before Going Out

A little planning can help. Have a real meal before you leave so you won't be tempted by the bread basket.

Try:

- Protein + fat combo: Eggs + avocado, or ground beef with sweet potato

- Add a sprinkle of sea salt to support hydration
- Avoid sugar spikes and crashes that mess with your glow

Restaurant Swaps That Still Slap

You're not packing your dressing, but you can make better choices without being the difficult one at the table.

- Swap seed oil salad dressings for olive oil + lemon or vinegar
- Ask for butter instead of "vegetable oil" on your side dishes
- Choose grilled over fried, but don't panic over a few truffle fries
- Order a protein-forward meal and build from there

Yes, restaurants cook with seed oils. Yes, it's annoying. But worrying about it does more harm than a few crispy potatoes ever could.

The Morning After: No Shame, Just Strategy

Glow girls don't punish. We uplift.

Here's how to recover without falling apart:

- Re-Lyte or sea salt water first thing in the morning.
- Eat real food early: protein plus fat, no sugary stuff.

- Go outside for 15 minutes with sunglasses on (no one will know).
- Lymphatic support: dry brushing, gua sha, or gentle stretching.
- No guilt. Just care.

Glow Girl Weekend Recap

Here's your checklist to maintain the glow intensity through Sunday night:

Glow Habit	Done?
Salt + lemon water	
Ate before going out	
Selected a healthier cocktail/mocktail.	
Moved the next morning	
Ordered what I wanted—and didn't spiral over it.	

Weekly Affirmation

"I can go out, have fun, eat fries, and still glow the next day—because joy and wellness aren't enemies."

Chapter 5: Glow with the Flow

Glow From the Inside Out

Here's the part no one talks about: glowing isn't just about SPF, truffle fries, or cute gym sets. It's about your nervous system and your energy levels. The version of you that wakes up and decides how the day will go, even before you open Instagram.

Let's be honest. You can have the perfect breakfast and spiral by noon if your stress is high and your nervous system is exhausted. That's not failure. It's a sign: your body needs support, not criticism.

We all do it: scroll past a "soft life" morning routine, feel inspired for two minutes, then snap at someone because your nervous system is barely holding on. This chapter is your toolkit for feeling grounded again, without needing a spa or 90 minutes of silence.

First Glow Truth: Calm Is a Skill

You weren't born frazzled. You were trained to be that way. And now, we're working on untraining it.

A regulated nervous system isn't about being Zen 24/7. It's about returning to calm faster, easier, and without spiraling. Start with these:

- Splashing cold water on your face can even reset your vagus nerve.
- Weighted blanket or body pressure (stimulates serotonin).
- Take slow exhales (inhale for 4 seconds, exhale for 6 seconds).
- Put your phone down — yes, even for just 10 minutes.

You don't need an entire "routine." What you need are reminders that you're safe.

Micro-Rituals for Boosting Mood (Under 2 Minutes)

These aren't just feel-good tricks. They're science-backed methods to change your mood quickly.

- Magnesium spray or bath flakes (your nervous system absorbs it)
- Touch grass—literally. Or hug a tree. Or water your plants barefoot.
- Light an essential oil candle (lavender, citrus, or eucalyptus).
- Flip through a real magazine (nostalgia = therapy).
- Stand in the sun—even if only for 30 seconds.
- Hug yourself (sounds silly, works wonders)

Glow isn't only what people see. It's what you feel.

Reminder: Moving Still Helps Reset Your Mood

Movement isn't just about fitness — it's about flow. You already have your daily walk and mini workout routine from earlier chapters. Now it's time to integrate it with your mood rituals.

You don't need to add anything more. Keep stacking the glow.

Glow Girl Dual Tracker

One part movement. One part mindset. Both parts shining.

Daily Glow Checklist	Mon Tue Wed Thu Fri
Morning stretch or walk	
Cold water or ice face dip	
Touch grass (yes, really)	
Phone break (10+ min)	
Light a candle or read a magazine.	
Magnesium or salt water	

Complete 4 out of 6? You've earned your Inner Reset + Outer Movement Glow Badge.

What to Do When You Feel Off

Say this out loud: *"Nothing is wrong with me. Something needs support."*

Then pick one:

- Drink salted lemon water.
- Lie on the floor like a Victorian ghost.
- Put your legs up the wall
- Text someone who makes you feel seen
- Open this book (you knew I was gonna say it)

You're not being dramatic. You're experiencing dysregulation. And this chapter is your comeback guide.

Weekly Affirmation

"I regulate my nervous system like a pro—cold water, cheekbone lifts, and disappearing into the backyard barefoot like a hot woodland fairy."

Chapter 6: Clean Girl Era

The Glow-Up Guide: Skin, Hair, and a Little Delusion

You know the feeling. You start to check the weather, and 20 minutes later, you've watched six Reels on "the only three concealers you'll ever need," two get-ready-with-me GRWMs, and a makeup fridge restock tour that somehow makes you question your whole bathroom drawer.

Beauty content is everywhere—and honestly, it's fun. The slow-motion makeup application, clever transitions, and the subtle nod to "clean girl aesthetic" mixed with glitter and full glam. You find yourself thinking: Do I need another foundation? Is that cheek contour going to change my life? But here's the thing: most of what's trending is toxic. Literally.

Many "holy grail" products are filled with fragrance, hormone-disrupting preservatives, and microplastics. That drugstore dupe everyone swears by? Likely tested on rabbits and coated in endocrine disruptors.

Fragrance: The Vibe That Lies

"Fragrance" sounds innocent, like a fresh linen candle or a pink sparkly lip gloss. But on a label, it's code for: "we don't have to tell you what's in here." It's a legal loophole that allows over 3,000 hidden chemicals to hide under one word. Some of these are known allergens, hormone disruptors, immune irritants, or carcinogens—and companies aren't required to list a single one.

Fragrance can throw off your endocrine system, mess with your estrogen, and worsen symptoms like fatigue, skin rashes, headaches, and brain fog. One swipe of "vanilla shimmer" can send your body into inflammation mode without you ever realizing it. And no—"unscented" doesn't always mean fragrance-free. Sometimes it just means another masking agent was added.

You wouldn't eat something with mystery ingredients. Don't let your skin drink it in either.

We're not here to age prematurely or harm our glow from the inside just for five seconds of aesthetic satisfaction.
So, we're approaching it differently.
This chapter is about beauty that feels good on your skin and conscience. We'll keep the fun—skip the hidden toxins. You can still master your glow, slicked-back ponytail, and lashes long enough to cast a shadow look. We just read the ingredients first.

And if you feel like throwing on red lipstick and vanishing into a metaphorical forest because your reputation has never been worse? Girl, same. Let's make it look intentional.

Skin First, Always

Your makeup looks its best when the skin underneath is healthy. We don't need perfection but want clarity, hydration, and bounce.

Glow Girl Skincare Basics:

- Double cleanse at night, especially if you're wearing SPF or makeup
- Use a mineral-based sunscreen, always zinc-based, with no exceptions
- Avoid fragrances in products that remain on your skin
- Read your labels: if you can't pronounce it, pause before applying
- Hydrate with aloe, rosewater mist, or a simple hyaluronic serum

Remember: glowing skin doesn't crack under pressure—or foundation.

Makeup Without the Mayhem

Here's your Glow Mode-approved starter kit, a lineup of everyday swaps I use and love. Before you dive in, just one thing: always patch test new products first. Everyone's skin is different, and your glow should never come with irritation.

That said, it's worth peeking at the ingredient list of what you're already using. Many popular products are loaded with hormone disruptors, sneaky synthetic fillers, and marketing fluff. The stuff we're tossing? Petroleum-packed lip goop, talc-heavy powders, and mascaras that sound like pharmaceutical ads.

What we're reaching for instead:

• Tinted mineral SPF (because foundation is out, and zinc is in)
• Cream blush + highlighter (bonus if it glows with mica, not talc)
• Paraben-free brow gel (fluffy and safe)
• Mascara that doesn't require a PhD to decode the label
• Lip oil or balm with real oils, not lab-made gloss
• Vitamin C serum (*Glow Tip: Your Vitamin C Serum

Shouldn't Read Like a Recipe Book)

• Whipped tallow (your skin's new BFF—promise)

*When you're shopping for a real Vitamin C serum, flip that label. If it looks like a grocery list with 50+ ingredients you can't pronounce, put it back. Clean, effective Vitamin C serum usually has fewer than 10 ingredients. Here's what *actually matters*:

- L-Ascorbic Acid (or another stable form like Sodium Ascorbyl Phosphate): This is the real Vitamin C—look for it high on the list.
- Water or Aloe Base: A good serum typically begins with water, aloe, or a combination of both.
- Ferulic Acid + Vitamin E (Tocopherol): These help stabilize Vitamin C and boost its effectiveness.
- No fragrance, dyes, or silicones: These are unnecessary and can irritate your skin or clog pores.

These aren't must-haves. They're glow-haves. Start slow. Swap one. See how you feel. And remember, what's in your glow bag matters as much as what's in your snack drawer.

Do you *need* a 14-step contour routine? No. Do you want to try it sometimes because it feels theatrical and fun? Absolutely. But always read the label before you glam.

My AM Routine (a.k.a. Why People Think I'm Aging Backward, Possibly a Vampire, or Enrolled in Hogwarts Night School for Skincare)

Before the school drop-off line even sees my face, I've already dabbed on a vitamin C serum that smells like citrus ambition, slathered on a zinc SPF that leaves zero white cast, and stood in front of my red light panel like a wellness warrior summoning her glow.

Is it a lot? Not really. Is it effective? Let's say I'm asked *"what I use"* more often than *"what I do."*

These are the ride-or-dies:

- Vitamin C serum (because dullness isn't a vibe)
- Zinc-based SPF (for sun protection, not a chemical cocktail)
- Non-LED Red light therapy (my face's version of morning coffee)
- Ice roller or ice cube face dunk (because I woke up puffy and unbothered)
- Relyte and coffee (because I've evolved—but I'm not insane)

It's not a 27-step routine—just a few glow-hacks I'd group-text you about. Because "you're glowing" is the best compliment, and I want you to hear it, too. I know you're all wondering whether I get Botox. Haven't gone there yet. It turns out that tallow and sleep are doing the job, for now. Not because I'm here to shame anyone, but because I have personal reservations about what's in some injectables (yes, I read ingredient lists for syringes too). I believe in letting people make their own choices—this book shows you what's also possible. I'm also opting for the natural route, as long as it still works. This routine isn't a dig at anyone opting for injectables—it's a glow-up guide for those who want to see how far skin, sleep, tallow, and zinc can take them. These aren't instant-fix tricks, but they work slowly, surely, and with fewer forehead freeze moments. Consistent habits, clean products, and the right glow make strangers ask what serum you use. (Spoiler: it's all listed above.)

Hair That Looks Expensive (Without the Drama)
You don't need a Dyson Airwrap or a 75-minute blowout.
You need:

- A clarifying shampoo (use once a week to detox your follicles)

- A silk pillowcase (or satin bonnet)
- Castor oil or rosemary oil for hair growth
- Less heat styling, more slick-back styles
- Slick your hair back with castor oil, twist it high, and tie it tight—instant cheekbone lift, no appointment needed.

Glow Moments Worth Romanticizing

Romanticize your beauty routine as if it's your second job:

- Wash your face while music plays
- Store your products in cute glass jars or small trays
- Turn your moisturizer into a face massage
- Use cold rollers or spoons in the morning
- Set your look with mineral mist and say, "She's ready for her reputation era" (wink)

You're not high-maintenance—you're high glow.

Weekly Affirmation

"I glow like I own the record-breaking tour of my life—and my SPF is non-toxic."

This Just In
(AND THAT'S JUST OUT)

WHAT'S IN	WHAT'S OUT
BEING THE MAIN CHARACTER IN YOUR OWN LIFE	PERFORMING FOR THE ALGORITHM
WIRED HEADPHONES (RETRO AND EMF-FRIENDLY)	AIRPODS IN EVERY ORIFICE
RED LIGHT MASKS & ICE ROLLERS	$300 FACIALS WITH ZERO FOLLOW-UP
10-MINUTE HOME WORKOUTS WITH SOUP CANS	"NO DAYS OFF" HUSTLE ENERGY
ZINC-BASED SPF & CASTOR OIL SLICK-BACKS	FRAGRANCE-LOADED 'DEWY GLOW' LIES
ACTUAL BOOKS AND MAGAZINES	47 TABS OF HALF-READ ARTICLES
TALLOW BALM & BAR SOAP	19-STEP SKINCARE ROUTINES YOU DON'T EVEN LIKE
CLEAN GIRL, SOFT GIRL, YOUR GIRL	COPY-PASTE INFLUENCERS
RE-LYTE, SEA SALT, AND SIPPING WATER LIKE IT'S A COCKTAIL	GUZZLING PLAIN WATER AND WONDERING WHY YOU'RE STILL DEHYDRATED
ORDERING A MATCHA WITH COCONUT MILK AND ZERO PUMPS	6-PUMP CARAMEL MACCHIATO PRETENDING TO BE HEALTHY
AGREEING TO DISAGREE, WITH STYLE	SCREAMING ON THE INTERNET
INDEPENDENT POLITICAL PODCASTERS WITH ACTUAL NUANCE	MAINSTREAM MEDIA RAGE BAIT
A LITTLE DELUSION + A LOT OF DISCERNMENT	BEING CYNICAL AND CALLING IT "REALISM"
SCREEN TIME LIMITS (SET BY YOU)	DOOMSCROLLING LIKE IT'S CARDIO
WALKING IN SILENCE FOR THE DRAMA	TRAUMA-DUMPING ON STORIES
KNOWING YOUR CYCLE AND SYNCING YOUR LIFE	WHITE-KNUCKLING YOUR LUTEAL PHASE WITH ICED COFFEE
HEALING YOUR GUT, NOT JUST YOUR TIKTOK FEED	GASLIGHT, GATEKEEP, GIRLBOSS (SHE'S TIRED)
QUIET LUXURY ENERGY WITH A COSTCO BUDGET	$80 CANDLES THAT SMELL LIKE REGRET
GLOWING AND LOGGING OFF	FAKING PEACE FOR THE ALGORITHM

Chapter 7: Clutter? I Don't Know Her.

Clean Your Space, Clear Your Mind

Have you ever scrolled past one of those "Sunday Reset" Reels where someone in a beige set glides through her spotless home with a cordless vacuum and an oat milk latte? It looks soothing. You save it, thinking, "I could be her." Then you look around at your exploded diaper bag, three Amazon boxes, and a chair that's more laundry pile than furniture—and you close the app.

Let's be honest: real resets don't look like that. However, they can feel even better.

You need space to think because you don't need a matching set or a designer mop. You need a vibe that supports you, not overwhelms you. And that begins with less stuff—and more peace.

The Real Glow Clean Philosophy

This chapter isn't about perfection. It's about making space—physically and mentally. A cluttered house makes your brain feel noisy. It keeps your cortisol high and your motivation low. A clean, calm space? It whispers, "You've got this."

So here's what's out:

- Buying every new "learning toy" for your kid that ends up under the couch
- Letting *any* store's "seasonal steals" turn into future clutter
- Decluttering 18 rooms in one day, crashing, and then resenting your house

What's in?

- Clearing one surface. One drawer. One space at a time.
- Letting go of things that stress you out just by existing.
- Remembering that *you don't have to keep things just because you paid for them.*

Less stuff means more clarity, fewer decisions, and more calm.

The Glow Room Reset: One Room at a Time

We go room by room—because glow doesn't happen in a panic.

Bedroom

The Rule: Only items that bring peace should be on your nightstand.

- Swap clutter for a candle, a book, and a water glass
- Put laundry away while watching your favorite comfort show
- Add a few drops of lavender to your pillow (you'll sleep deeper, promise)

Kitchen

The Rule: Clear counters = clear mind

- Do the dishes while listening to a good podcast
- Toss expired food without guilt
- Wipe surfaces with a non-toxic spray.
- *Bonus glow:* Lemon peels in a simmer pot = instant spa vibes

Bathroom

The Rule: If it's crusty, dusty, or smells like a chemistry lab, it goes

- Say farewell to 2017 mascara
- Clean using baking soda, vinegar, and essential oils.
- Refill towels and Q-tips as if you're managing a cozy Airbnb.

Living Room

The Rule: Cozy, not chaotic

- One bin or basket for kids' stuff
- Fold blankets, fluff pillows, and light a candle.
- Vacuum as if you're on a mission to impress only yourself.

Laundry

The Rule: Romanticize the chore

- Fold laundry while watching a comfort show or an old rom-com.
- Play music, light incense, and spray linen mist.
- Reward yourself afterward. You deserve it.

Touch Grass (Yes, Literally)

Once your space feels more peaceful, go outside. Allow sunlight and soil to refresh your energy. Walk barefoot in the yard, water your plants, and take three deep breaths. You're not lazy or overwhelmed. You're just too indoors and overstimulated. Let the ground bring you back.

Your Glow Clean Tracker

Room	Reset This Week? (Y/N)
Bedroom	
Kitchen	
Bathroom	
Living Room	
Laundry	
Touch Grass	

Do what you can. Don't aim for spotlessness—aim for sanity.

Weekly Affirmation

"I get judged enough by Instagram moms and my reflection—I don't need my house judging me as well."

Chapter 8: Fashion Haul? More Like Emotional Baggage Claim

The Confidence Closet

Instagram is obsessed with hauls. Hauls from H&M, hauls from Zara, and hauls from "random Amazon brands you've never heard of but suddenly need to own." It's nonstop. And if you're not careful, you end up with five versions of the same top and no outfits that feel good.

Let's break that cycle.

This chapter isn't about following trends. It's about creating a wardrobe that supports you. Clothes that fit, enhance, and boost your confidence—without bursting out of your drawers or whispering guilt trips every morning.

Stop Letting Your Closet Gaslight You

Ever open your closet, look at the jam-packed racks, and still think, "I have nothing to wear"? Same.

That's not your fault—it's decision fatigue.

A cluttered closet can deceive you:

- "You spent money on this, so you should keep it."
- "It doesn't fit now, but maybe it will."
- "It's trendy... right?"

45

We're done letting hangers guilt-trip us—it's time to refresh.

The Hanger Flip Rule

It's clever. It's straightforward. And it reveals the truth.

- Flip every hanger in your closet backward.
- Every time you wear something, rehang it normally.
- After 6–12 months, anything still hanging backward? Donate it.

If you didn't wear it in real life, then it's not truly your style.

How to Know If You Need It

Ask yourself:

- Would I repurchase this today?
- Do I feel good when I wear it?
- Is this about a version of me that's no longer me?
- Am I doing this out of guilt or excitement?

The goal isn't to have fewer clothes but fewer regrets.

Closet Staples That Don't Go Out of Style

When in doubt, stick to classic styles. These glow girl essentials will take you season after season without a total identity crisis.

• A well-fitting pair of jeans (not the ones that haunt you)

- A crisp white T-shirt
- A black or neutral blazer
- A slip dress or a midi that makes you feel expensive
- A leather (or faux) jacket
- Great sunglasses
- Nude and black shoes that go with everything
- Gold hoops or minimal jewelry
- A bag that fits your real life (diapers? laptop? both?)

Keep these. Build around them. They're the opposite of impulse shopping hauls.

Budget Closet Glow-Up: Small Upgrades, Big Confidence

You don't need a walk-in or a capsule wardrobe. Instead, focus on these simple wins:

- Match your hangers—all black, all white—clean and cohesive.
- Clip hangers—for matching sets, skirts, or just pretending you run a boutique.
- Add a bin or two—one for lounge, one for "don't know where it goes," and one for "donate soon."
- Fix the lighting—even a $10 motion light strip makes your closet feel like a grown woman lives here.
- Weekly outfit rack—pick 3–5 outfits ahead of time. Done.

• Confidence shelf—for your perfume, your claw clips, and your "I'm that girl" earrings.

A Closet That Matches *You*

You are not here to shrink to fit old jeans.

You're here to get dressed in under five minutes, feel great, and enjoy your life.

Glow Mode Hack: Color Analysis 101

Ever wonder why some outfits make you look effortlessly radiant, while others just feel...off? That's the magic (and science) of seasonal color analysis.

Based on your skin undertone, natural hair, and eye color, you fall into a "season" like **True Winter**, **Soft Autumn**, or **Light Spring**. Each season has a color palette that complements your features, making you look radiant, refreshed, and effortlessly stylish.

The right colors = skin glows, eyes sparkle, zero effort.
The wrong ones = dull, washed-out, or like you need under-eye concealer when you don't.

Curious where your glow lives? Take our mini Glow Palette Quiz and uncover your signature season—because some colors were always meant for you.

What's your seasonal color match? Let's find out what brings out your glow.

1. What happens when you stand in direct sunlight?

A. I tan quickly and deeply

B. I burn easily, then fade to pink or fair

C. I burn *and* tan (it's complicated)

D. I don't tan—I freckle or stay pale

---

2. Look at your veins in natural light. What color do they appear?

A. Greenish

B. Bluish or purple

C. A mix—I can't tell

D. Neutral/olive

---

3. Which jewelry makes your skin look more radiant?

A. Gold

49

B. Silver

C. Rose gold or mixed metals

D. Depends on the outfit

---

4. What kind of colors do you naturally gravitate toward?

A. Warm, earthy tones like camel, olive, terracotta

B. Cool, bold tones like black, royal blue, icy pink

C. Muted pastels and soft neutrals

D. Bright, punchy colors like coral, teal, or hot pink

---

5. What best describes your natural coloring?

A. Medium to dark hair, warm-toned skin, golden or hazel eyes

B. Light skin, high contrast (dark hair + light eyes OR light hair + dark eyes)

C. Soft/blended—nothing really stands out (hair, skin, and eyes are similar)

D. Cool-toned skin with medium features and soft eyes (gray, blue, or soft brown)

Your Results:

Mostly A's – You're a Warm Glow Girl (Autumn/Spring):
You shine in **warm, golden tones**—think copper, mustard, cream, olive, and coral. Earth tones bring out your radiance. Gold jewelry is your BFF.

Mostly B's – You're an Icy Icon (True/Cool Winter):
Your look pops in **cool, crisp colors** like navy, fuchsia, pure white, and emerald. Avoid warm shades—they dull your sparkle. Silver suits you best.

Mostly C's – You're a Soft Glow Girl (Soft Autumn or Summer):
You look stunning in **muted tones**—dusty rose, sage, periwinkle, and stone. Keep it low-contrast. Think linen neutrals, delicate pastels, and creamy textures.

Mostly D's – You're a Bold Glow Babe (Clear/Bright Spring or Winter):
You light up in **saturated brights**—electric blue, lemon yellow, cherry red. Go for contrast and clarity. You wear color like confidence.

Weekly Affirmation

"I dress for the woman I am today—and she deserves hangers that match, pants that fit, and clothes that hype her up, not haunt her."

Chapter 9: Screen Time Called. I Declined.

The Digital Detox You Want to Do

You set a 15-minute timer on Instagram.

It pops up.

You hit "Ignore." Three times.

Then suddenly it's 11:47 PM, and you're watching a stranger in Belgium organize her fridge with rainbow-coded produce while you have half a string cheese and a questionable cucumber in yours.

We've all been there. You start with good intentions—just checking DMs or seeing what your college roommate's cousin wore to her baby shower. But five scrolls in, you're annoyed, overstimulated, and subtly spiraling over a life that's not yours. It's not just social media. It's the tabs, the apps, the doomscrolling, and the constant need to stay productive, connected, and aesthetically evolved. Here's the truth: Your brain is begging for a break.

The Glow Detox Approach

We're not deleting everything or going off-grid. (Though we enjoy that idea.) We're making intentional swaps—small changes that safeguard your mental space and help you regain control of your energy.

Because your glow? She doesn't live on your phone.

How to Take a Break (Without Losing Your Mind)

Try one. Try them all. Repeat what works.

- Delete the apps for the weekend. You can re-download them on Monday. (Spoiler: You won't miss anything.)
- Put your phone in another room during meals. It's like it's 2006.
- Switch to grayscale mode to make scrolling less addictive and appealing. As a bonus, wear blue-light glasses.
- Charge your phone in another room at night. EMFs are real; you'll sleep better when your nervous system isn't pinging like a group chat.
- Replace morning scrolling with something tactile: a page of a book, a journal entry, stretching, or simply staring at the ceiling like it's a wellness ritual.
- Set a "closing shift." One hour before bed, no screens. We're not baristas, but we *are* resetting the vibe.

What to Do With All That Extra Time

You'll be shocked how much brain space returns when you're not constantly stimulated.

Ideas:

- Light an essential oil candle and fold laundry to a good movie
- Go analog: read a magazine, write a letter, touch grass (literally)
- Call someone. Yes, on the phone. Bonus points if it's your mom, grandma, or favorite aunt
- Take a hot girl walk without documenting it
- Make your skincare routine last a little longer
- Play music while you clean one room. Just one. That's enough
- Daydream. (It's not lazy—it's brain yoga)

You know it. You've lived in it and scrolled through it.
It's the silent sentence we serve every time we believe the next thing will fix us. The next outfit. The next "That Girl" vacation spot. The next filtered version of someone else's life.

But it runs deeper than just products or posts.
Life seems complete on paper—marriage, home, family—yet the desire for something more refuses to be satisfied... as if joy exists in the next thing instead of the present moment.

That's the *Jail of Want.*

This book felt complete—until I heard something at Mass that stopped me in my tracks. Our priest spoke about "The Jail of Want," and I knew I had to come back and share it with you.

Built from comparison. Fueled by discontent. Locked by the lie that what you have—who you are—isn't enough.

But here's your release: Gratitude is the key.
You don't need more to be whole. You need to remember how to want less.

So shut the app. Unsubscribe from the fantasy. The glow you're chasing? It's already in you. You just forgot how bright it was without the noise. This isn't your usual affirmation. It's something more—a reminder straight from me to you, because this one couldn't be left unsaid.

You've been lied to—about looks, likes, and labels.
Social media trained you to crave hearts on a screen and praise from people you'll never meet.

But likes aren't legacy.
Filters aren't reality.
And glow doesn't come from comparison—it comes from clarity.

In the real world? The algorithm isn't the standard.
Confidence is.

Maybe the biggest glow-up of all...is realizing you were never missing anything to begin with.

XOXO,
Margot

Chapter 10: Don't Rush Me—I'm Romanticizing My Errands

The Soft Life Schedule (Without Quitting Your Job)

You've seen the reels: slow mornings, matcha lattes, quiet walks in matching outfits, a voiceover whispering "I no longer hustle—I attract."

Beautiful. Inspiring. A little unhinged.

Because for most of us, the soft life doesn't come with a content team or a trust fund. You're either chasing toddlers, chasing deadlines, or just seeking a little peace amid everything else.

This chapter is for women who want to feel calmer without comparing themselves to the perfectly edited morning routines of influencers—or even their best friends, who have fewer responsibilities and more time to journal in linen pajamas.

Whether you're 24 and overwhelmed by hustle culture, 34 and quietly burning out from trying to do it all, or 44 and standing at the edge of your prime, *setting fresh goals, chasing long-postponed passions, or stepping into a season that's hers alone—* **this chapter is your gentle permission slip:** *to breathe, rest, and build a soft life that suits you.*

You don't need Bali. You need breathing room.

What Soft Looks Like *For You*

The soft life isn't about luxury. It's about *lightness*. A softer schedule means:

- More flow, less force
- Saying no without writing a 12-paragraph apology text
- Finding 15 quiet minutes without needing permission
- Not rushing through your own life like you're late to something

It's the pause before the scroll, the walk before the rant, the exhale before the reply.

Build Your Soft Schedule

You don't need to overhaul your calendar—shift a few things with intention.

1. Create Bookends to Your Day

- Morning: Wake up 10 minutes earlier to sit in silence. Not to scroll. Not to clean. Just sit.
- Night: Light a candle. Write something you're proud of. Brush your hair gently, not quickly.

2. Buffer Everything by 5 Minutes

Running late = panic. Permit yourself to *arrive*. Add five minutes between calls, pickups, appointments, and even dinner. That's a soft buffer.

3. Schedule "Nothing"

Schedule 30 minutes on your calendar and mark it as "Nothing." Guard it, defend it, and intentionally keep it unproductive.

4. Romanticize the Boring Stuff

- Laundry? Light a candle and play old jazz.
- Dishes? Try a guided meditation while you do them.
- Email? Diffuse peppermint oil and wear a robe. Power move.

This is your life. Make it nice.

5. Ask Yourself This Daily

What's the most caring thing I can do for myself today?
Even if the answer is just "put on socks and drink water," that still counts.

Normalize the *Affordable* Soft Life

You don't need a $200 spa day. Try:

- A DIY oil scalp massage while watching your comfort show

- Magnesium bath + candle = instant nervous system reset
- Saying no to an event you're dreading = free peace
- Switching your phone to Airplane Mode = luxury

Soft isn't about money. It's about *margin*.

Weekly Affirmation

"I loosen my schedule, not my standards. Peace is powerful. Rest is revolutionary. And I get to set my own rules."

Chapter 11: Aisle Be Glowing

The Glow Girl Grocery Cart

You open TikTok "just to check one thing" and suddenly find yourself deep into someone's $400 Trader Joe's haul, with ten types of pickled vegetables, five imported cheeses, and a bag of cinnamon-dusted almonds you've never seen at your store before. At first, you're inspired. Then, you're spiraling—Googling adaptogens, adding niche snacks to cart, and wondering if you've failed at wellness because your pantry doesn't look like a cottagecore mood board. Let's stop that cycle right now.

In Chapter 3, we kept it simple. You learned the basics—easy meal ideas, glow-friendly habits, and a few snack swaps—and that was your starting point. Now? This is your upgrade. The list you screenshot. The guide you keep handy. The one you carry around while trying to ignore the "seasonal aisle" that somehow makes you want to buy a third jar of maple-flavored mustard.

We're talking real food. No seed oils. Affordable alternatives. And yes—organic where it matters. Because your food should nourish you, not make you wonder what glyphosate is doing to your insides.

FYI: Some people—smart, vocal, persistent—are working behind the scenes to hold companies accountable for what they put in our food. Be glad they exist. And remember: *Health isn't partisan. It's personal.*

Let's fill your cart the way the glow girl you are.

Why Organic? Here's the Quick Tea:

Glyphosate (the chemical herbicide sprayed on many non-organic crops) has been linked to inflammation, gut issues, and hormone disruption. While not everything in your cart needs to be organic, choosing organic for the Dirty Dozen, oils, dairy, and animal products can make a real difference.

The Dirty Dozen (and yes, I'll handle the heavy lifting—because I know you're not about to Google it mid-read):

These fruits and vegetables tend to absorb the most pesticide residue, which you do not want in your smoothie. When possible, choose the organic versions of these and thank yourself later.

- Strawberries
- Spinach
- Kale, collard & mustard greens
- Grapes

- Peaches

- Pears

- Nectarines

- Apples

- Bell and hot peppers

- Cherries

- Blueberries

- Green beans

You don't need to be perfect—just aware. This is glow shopping, not guilt shopping.

Grocery Cart Staples

Here's your Glow Girl shopping list. Take a screenshot of it. Please print it out. Text it to yourself. Use it.

Glow Girl
SHOPPING LIST

PRODUCE
- LEMONS (MORNING LEMON WATER)
- SPINACH, ARUGULA, AND/OR MIXED GREENS
- AVOCADOS
- CUCUMBERS
- BERRIES (ORGANIC IF POSSIBLE)
- BANANAS OR APPLES
- FROZEN CAULIFLOWER RICE OR ZUCCHINI NOODLES
- SWEET POTATOES

PROTEINS
- EGGS (PASTURE-RAISED IF BUDGET ALLOWS)
- ORGANIC GROUND TURKEY, CHICKEN THIGHS, OR BEEF
- WILD-CAUGHT SALMON OR SARDINES
- COTTAGE CHEESE, GREEK YOGURT (FULL-FAT, NO ADDED SUGAR)
- BONE BROTH (OR MAKE YOUR OWN!)

FATS
- COCONUT OIL, GHEE, OR GRASS-FED BUTTER
- OLIVE OIL (ORGANIC, IN DARK GLASS BOTTLE)
- OLIVES
- CHEESE (BLOCK OR WEDGE FORM TO AVOID ADDITIVES)
- TAHINI (GREAT FOR DRESSINGS OR DIPS)

PANTRY PICKS
- CANNED BEANS (RINSE BEFORE USING)
- RICE, QUINOA, OR LENTIL PASTA
- ORGANIC TOMATO SAUCE
- ALMOND FLOUR OR CASSAVA FLOUR
- CINNAMON, TURMERIC, GARLIC POWDER
- RAW HONEY OR MAPLE SYRUP (IN SMALL AMOUNTS!)

SNACKS THAT WON'T BETRAY YOU
- HARD-BOILED EGGS
- SEAWEED SNACKS
- COCONUT CHIPS
- MEDJOOL DATES TOPPED WITH A TOUCH OF ALMOND BUTTER
- CHEESE CUBES AND BERRIES

HYDRATION STATION
- RELYTE PACKETS (SALT-BASED ELECTROLYTES THAT HYDRATE YOU)
- SPRING OR FILTERED WATER
- HERBAL TEAS LIKE PEPPERMINT, GINGER, OR DANDELION ROOT.

THESE FRUITS AND VEGETABLES TEND TO ABSORB THE MOST PESTICIDE RESIDUE, WHICH YOU DO NOT WANT IN YOUR SMOOTHIE. WHEN POSSIBLE, CHOOSE THE ORGANIC VERSIONS OF THESE AND THANK YOURSELF LATER.

- STRAWBERRIES-SPINACH-KALE
- COLLARD & MUSTARD GREENS
- GRAPES, PEACHES, PEARS
- NECTARINES, APPLES
- BELL AND HOT PEPPERS
- CHERRIES, BLUEBERRIES
- GREEN BEANS

Pro Glow Tips:

- If it says "vegetable oil," put it back. End of story.
- Read ingredient labels—ignore them if they sound like a chemistry experiment.
- Shop the outer aisles first. That's where the best food is.
- If you wouldn't cook with it at home, don't eat it from a box.

Your Simple Weekly Glow Menu

No need for 45-minute recipes with 19 ingredients. Here's a simple framework to follow:

Breakfast:

Eggs + avocado + fruit

Or full-fat yogurt + berries + cinnamon

Lunch:

Big salad with protein, olives, and a simple oil + vinegar dressing

Or bone broth with leftover veggies + rice

Dinner:

Protein + roasted veg + small carb (sweet potato, rice, etc.)

Or stir-fry with coconut aminos over cauliflower rice

Snacks:

Real ones. See the snack list above. They exist for a reason.

Weekly Affirmation

"My grocery cart is my glow-up toolkit. I choose food that fuels me, not fakes me out."

Chapter 12: This Label's Got Trust Issues

Did we cover this already? Absolutely. But if food marketers can repeat their tricks, I can repeat the truth.

There's a reason health food marketing feels like a scam with a green juice filter. It kind of is. Labels know how to charm you: "all-natural," "heart-healthy," "pasture-raised," "no added hormones"—phrases that sound like truth but are basically vibes. Let's decode them.

You're standing in the aisle holding a bottle of dressing. It says "organic," "heart healthy," and "made with avocado oil."
You feel good. Until you flip it over and see... canola oil, sunflower oil, and something called "natural flavors."
Cue the spiral.
Welcome to the modern grocery store, where marketing is louder than facts, and the ingredient list is where the truth hides. This chapter is your decoder ring. Because let's be real: reading food labels isn't intuitive. It's exhausting, confusing, and sometimes downright sneaky.
Let's make it make sense.

The Front of the Label Lies (Most of the Time)

That bold "Non-GMO" or "All Natural" badge on the front? It's marketing, not science. The truth is only in the ingredients list and nutrition panel—and even those require decoding.

Here's the secret: you don't have to read everything. You just need to know what to focus on—and what to avoid like a toxic ex.

What You're Looking For

When scanning a label, check for:

- Oils: Avoid seed oils like canola, soybean, sunflower, safflower, corn, and grapeseed.

  → Better options include tallow, ghee, butter, coconut oil, or real olive oil (but be cautious—more on that below).

- Sugars: Watch out for sneaky names like dextrose, maltodextrin, cane juice, and brown rice syrup. If it ends in "-ose," you probably don't need it.

- Additives & Fillers: Items like carrageenan, gums (xanthan, guar), "natural flavors," and "yeast extract" often mean: "we used science to make this taste good instead of food."

- Protein bars, snack packs, and 'health drinks': These are often the biggest culprits. Flip before you sip or bite.

What the Buzzwords *Really* Mean

Label Term	What It Really Means
"All Natural"	Meaningless. There's no legal standard.
"Heart Healthy"	It usually includes seed oils and whole grains, aka the inflammation duo.
"Non-GMO"	Good start, but it doesn't mean organic.
"Organic"	Better—but still check the complete list. You can have organic cane sugar and organic garbage.
"Made with Olive Oil"	Translation: *some* olive oil, canola, sunflower, and friends.

How to Spot a Good Product (Fast)

- Short list

  Five ingredients or fewer is a good start.

- You recognize everything

  If you can picture it in your kitchen, that's a win.

- It doesn't scream at you

  Products that brag *too much* often have something

  to hide.

Quick Rule of Thumb: Would My Great-Grandma Know What This Is?

If you need a degree in chemistry to understand it, it's probably not food.

The Olive Oil Conspiracy (Yes, It's Real)

Most olive oil on grocery store shelves is adulterated—aka cut with cheaper oils—even if it says "extra virgin."

Look for:

- Dark glass bottles
- Harvest and bottling dates
- Certifications like COOC or PDO

Or skip the drama and go with butter. Your brain will thank you.

The Glow Mode Label Test

Next time you pick something up, ask:

- Does it pass the oil test?
- Do I know what these ingredients are?

- Can I pronounce everything here?
- Does this support my glow, or is it just marketing to it?

Label Check Alert:
You read food labels—start reading your bathroom ones too. Bleached tampons and toilet paper can contain residues you don't want anywhere near your body. Choose organic or unbleached instead.

Weekly Affirmation:
"I don't fall for buzzwords. I read the label, trust my gut, and glow like a woman who knows what's in her food."

Chapter 13: Cutting You Off Looks Good on Me

Protect Your Peace, Protect Your Glow

You've cleaned out your pantry. You've read your labels. You're glowing up from the inside out. But there's one thing left—and it might be the most important: the people and pressures around you.

Let's talk about the real glow killers.

You're doing lemon water and magnesium mocktails, and someone says, "Wow, must be nice to have all that time." Or you're out to dinner with friends, feeling proud of your week of walks and seed-oil-free snacks, and you casually ask the server, "Do you cook with olive oil or vegetable oil?" Suddenly, the table goes silent, as if you have just asked for the blood type of the chef.

Yeah, I've changed. That's the point.

This chapter is your permission slip to stop shrinking yourself to fit anyone else's expectations. If your glow-up makes people uncomfortable, that's their work, not yours.

You Can't Glow Around People Who Drain You

You're allowed to set boundaries. You're allowed to say no. You can glow louder, stronger, and clearer—especially when someone tries to dim your light.

75

If someone makes fun of your zinc SPF, walk schedule, or clean deodorant, you don't owe them a TED Talk. Just smile, sip your electrolyte-infused water, and carry on. Wellness isn't a performance. It's a personal practice.

Sometimes, the most challenging part of growing up is realizing who doesn't support you. It's not always strangers online. It's your coworker who is cutting comments. Your best friend who suddenly acts weird when you order real food. The family member who says, "You're too much" when you're finally comfortable being yourself. That hurts. But it also sets you free.

You don't need everyone's approval to feel good in your life. You're not here to make others comfortable with your growth. You're here to take care of yourself. To glow up in a way that's honest, sustainable, and unapologetically yours. Your boundaries won't threaten the right people—they'll respect them. And the ones who don't? They're just not on your frequency anymore.

Sometimes, the person dimming your glow is yourself. You scroll through reels of women with glass skin, spotless kitchens, and gym routines that start at 5 a.m., and all of a sudden, your real life feels messy and behind. But you're not behind. You're living. And no one's highlight reel can match your true growth. Give yourself credit. You're doing more than enough—and you're allowed to shine even in the chaos.

The Not-So-Toxic Daily Routine

We understand—everything seems "toxic" these days. The internet can make you feel like even your toothpaste is out to get you. So, let's keep it simple. Here's a one-day routine with easy swaps you can make.

Time of Day	Old Routine	Glow Swap
Wake-up	Scroll phone in bed	Open the blinds, breathe deeply
Deodorant	Drugstore antiperspirant	Aluminum-free stick or go bare
Coffee	Oat milk creamer	Raw milk or coconut cream
Shower	Scented body wash	Fragrance-free or essential oil-based
Cleaning up	Bleach spray	Vinegar + lemon oil mix
Skincare	12-step trend routine	3-step real glow setup

Time of Day	Old Routine	Glow Swap
Haircare	Dry shampoo overload	Apple cider rinse + scalp oil
Evening unwind	Wine + phone scroll	Magnesium mocktail + good book
Night charging	Phone on nightstand	Phone in another room (EMF break!)

No pressure to do it all at once. Just pick one and start. You don't have to fix your whole life by Tuesday—you have to start protecting your peace like it's part of your skincare routine.

Weekly Affirmation

"If it drains, dulls, or doubts me, I'm out. I protect my peace like it's my one good side in a group photo."

Interlude

Step Away from the Kitchen Scissors—Take This Quiz Instead

Because you're not allowed to cut bangs until you stop relating to that "this is fine" dog meme.

A break from the chapters to figure out your aesthetic.

You've Heard of Hot Girl Summer... But What's *Your* Glow Mode Era?

Let's set the scene: You're hydrated, using zinc SPF, and glowing like a disco ball at golden hour. You've made it through the label-reading, closet-clearing, mocktail-ordering part of the journey—and now it's time to discover who you are in your Glow Era.

Answer these 10 questions quickly. No overthinking. Just go with your gut.

---

1. Your ideal Saturday morning starts with:

A) Ice face bath, lemon water, and blasting old-school jazz

B) A long walk, a coconut milk latte in hand, and a cute outfit to match

C) Organizing your fridge while listening to a political podcast

D) Sleeping in with a silk eye mask and ignoring the group chat

2. Your favorite wellness flex is:

A) Your DIY magnesium spray that smells like a spa

B) Your spotless fridge filled with prepped meals and fancy salts

C) Your non-toxic label knowledge that scares people (in a good way)

D) Your unmatched glow and mysterious cheekbone lift

3. Your energy right now is:

A) Guava Girl—soft, sweet, but with boundaries

B) Jam Girl—chaotic but romantic, thriving in the mess

C) Dolphin Girl—early riser, cold plunges, wears blue

D) Classic it-girl elegance, but with better ingredients

4. What's in your tote bag right now?

A) SPF stick, a journal, and a kombucha

B) Snacks, a vintage magazine, and rosewater spray

C) Grocery list, books with dog-eared pages, and magnesium drops

D) Silk scrunchie, tinted lip balm, and a linen napkin (just in case)

5. Your ultimate splurge is:

A) A full-body lymphatic drainage massage

B) A seasonal produce delivery box

C) A new water filter system

D) A blowout and high-thread-count sheets

6. You cry over:

A) A well-placed movie soundtrack

B) When your matcha froths just right

C) Environmental documentaries

D) A love letter you wrote to yourself (in your head)

7. Your lock screen is:

A) A photo of your dream kitchen or a vision board collage

B) Your dog, your kid, or a blurry beach sunset

C) An inspirational quote from a podcast

D) A black and white aesthetic selfie that hits

8. You decompress by:

A) Doing yoga in your living room with candles lit

B) Going on a Target run and coming home with only two extra things

C) Researching new ingredients while sipping tea

D) Rewatching your favorite movie for the 37th time

9. You feel most powerful when:

A) You speak your truth in a soft, strong way

B) You romanticize your to-do list

C) You educate someone with receipts

D) You walk into a room, and people notice your vibe before your outfit

10. Your dream text to receive is:

A) "Your skin looks incredible—what are you doing?"

B) "That mocktail recipe changed my life."

C) "You made me want to switch my deodorant."

D) "You're glowing. Whatever you're doing, it's working."

Tally It Up

Count how many A's, B's, C's, and D's you circled. Find your vibe below.

Mostly A's – You're a Glow Witch

You light candles with intention, make your tinctures, and you're the friend who always knows which aisle the good coconut oil is in. You create space for people to breathe more deeply.

Your song: *"Dog Days Are Over" by Florence + the Machine*

Mostly B's – Jam Girl Energy

You romanticize everything. Your laundry is folded to a soundtrack. Your dinners feel like summer in Provence. You're not here to be perfect but to live juicy.

Your song: *"August" by Taylor Swift*

Mostly Cs – Soft But Sharp

You care deeply and read everything. You're sending friends

non-toxic swap charts and educating the group chat with love (and receipts).

Your song: *"Ribs" by Lorde*

Mostly D's – Timeless Glow

Old soul. New tricks. You've curated a routine that feels more like a ritual, and you're never skipping mineral based SPF— even on cloudy days. Your glow speaks louder than your words.

Your song: *"Like a Girl" by Lizzo*

Chapter 14: We Are Not Gatekeeping This

Trending Tips, Tricks, and Products Worth Trying

You know how it goes. You see a video titled "I'm not gatekeeping this!" Thirty-eight seconds later, you're elbow-deep in a cart full of supplements, serums, or overnight oats in a jar. It's a lot.

Glow Mode isn't about pushing trends. It *is* about sharing what's actually worth trying—especially if it makes your life easier, more fun, or more radiant.

These are the things we like. Not because they're viral.

Because they work.

Holy Glow Grail

Products that go the extra mile without the extra toxins.

- Organic coconut oil is a versatile essential. It can serve as a moisturizer, makeup remover, hair mask, or oil pull for oral health. Plus, it smells like vacation.

- Chlorophyll drops: Add a few to your morning water for a skin boost.

    Tip: Choose a clean, reputable brand free of synthetic dyes or additives.

- Mineral-based deodorant: Begin with magnesium formulas if baking soda irritates your skin.

- Magnesium spray or flakes: Ideal for muscle recovery and better sleep. Spray on legs or add to your bath.
- Non-toxic dry brush: Supports lymphatic drainage and smooth skin.
  Tip: Brush toward your heart with long, upward strokes. Start at your feet and work your way up.

Glow Mode ON: Ageless and Irresistible
Little hacks that upgrade your routine—without upgrading your credit card balance.

- Kris Jenner ponytail lift (the non-surgical kind):
  Use a slick hair styling stick to create a clean, tight bun. Comb everything up, secure it, and remember the gold hoops.
- Red light therapy: Red light benefits skin health, mood, and mitochondria.
  Tip: If you're worried about LED exposure, opt for a non-LED red light panel. LED flicker and EMF can be irritating, so low-EMF, non-LED options are best if you're sensitive. Look for near-infrared, non-LED options that support collagen production and cellular repair.

- Silk pillowcases: Less frizz, fewer lines, and a feeling like a movie star.
- Cold rollers or chilled spoons: Keep them in the fridge for a de-puffing morning ritual.
- Face mists: Rose water, aloe, or mineral-rich thermal waters for a midday refresher.

Mom Hack, But Make It Chic

Gorgeous habits on autopilot.

- Applying a bentonite clay mask while folding laundry.
- Apply body oil before towel drying to lock in moisture.
- Spray magnesium on your shoulders while doing dishes.
- Put your laundry detergent in a pretty glass jar— because why not add a touch of romance?

Kitchen Counter Flex

Small swaps, big upgrades.

- Filtered water > tap water
- Coconut milk > oat milk
- Glass containers > plastic leftovers
- Organic eggs > "natural" claims

- Cast iron skillet > scratched-up nonstick
- Coffee with cinnamon > coffee with "natural flavors"

No Gatekeeping Allowed

You don't have to try everything. You don't even have to *buy* anything.

Glow Mode is more than just a concept; it's a way of life. It's about feeling good in your body and making smart choices about what you put in and on it. These tools? They're simply that—tools. Your glow was never in a bottle to start with. It's inside you, ready to be unleashed.

Weekly Affirmation

"I know the ingredients in my lotion, the intention behind my rituals, and the energy I bring into every room. My glow is not up for debate."

Chapter 15: TSA Took My Toner but Not My Glow

You swore you'd pack light. Just the essentials, right? Then suddenly you're at the gate with a duffel full of electrolyte packets, backup leggings, three kinds of snacks, and your travel-size red light device (because, yes, you are *that* girl now).

Travel doesn't have to interrupt your glow. Whether you're road-tripping to the lake, jetting off for a beach weekend, or attending a family reunion, this chapter is your glow-on-the-go game plan.

We're not about appearing perfect. We're about showing up prepared. So here's how to keep your mood steady, your skin calm, and your gut unbothered at 30,000 feet—or anywhere the GPS takes you.

Plane Mode, Activated

Air travel is dehydrating and draining, and it's full of mystery meals made with seed oils. But you? You've got a plan.

Glow Girl Flight Essentials:

- Organic snacks: Think seed-oil-free jerky, dark chocolate, cheese cubes, berries, and hard-boiled eggs in a cooler bag.

- Electrolyte tip: Water alone doesn't hydrate. Add a pinch of sea salt and a squeeze of lemon—or pack clean electrolyte packets like Re-Lyte.
- Zinc SPF and face mist: Cabin air is dry. Reapply mineral sunscreen and refresh your skin mid-flight.
- Silk eye mask and magnesium spray: Sleep is essential for a glow. To relax your muscles, spray magnesium oil on your legs or feet.
- Clean wipes and peppermint tea bags: for freshening up and soothing your stomach.
  Bonus move: Bring a small essential oil roller (lavender or peppermint) for a mid-flight mood boost.

Road Trip, But Make It Radiant

Your car = your wellness sanctuary on wheels. Skip the drive-thru. Stay in the zone.

Glow Girl Car Kit:
- Tote stocked with:
    - Organic gum or mints
    - Natural deodorant (Aluminum-free deodorant isn't niche anymore—check almost any shelf.)

- o Organic coconut oil (mini jar = all-purpose magic)
  - o Hair stick for flyaways and ponytail lifts
  - o Non-LED red light mini device if you're feeling luxe
- Movement: Stretch every 2–3 hours. Squats at the rest stop? Iconic.
- Fuel up right: Bring a portable cooler with organic grapes, coconut yogurt, clean protein bars, and sparkling water.
- Entertainment: Download your go-to podcast or audiobook. Bonus: Catch up on independent political voices instead of mainstream noise. Glow girl, but informed.

Must-Stop Pit Stops (Without Sabotage)

You're on the road, and someone *has* to stop at the gas station or fast-food spot. No problem.

Make the wise choice:

- Choose nuts, cheese sticks, plain jerky, or fruit over pastries and chips.
- Ask for no sauce or dressing at restaurants (or request it on the side).

- Stick to grilled over fried when you can.
- Drink water first—most road snacks are just thirst in disguise.

Dining with friends or family who didn't plan? Keep it flexible. You can ask about cooking oils or choose options without shame. One meal doesn't erase your glow, but it reminds you why you packed your snacks.

80/20 Glow Rule: Vacation Edition
No guilt. No restriction. Just intention.
Here's the mindset: 80% of the time, you nourish your body with what feels good long-term. 20% of the time, you eat the truffle fries, sip the cocktail, and live your life. You don't owe anyone perfection, not even yourself. The 80/20 Glow Rule is not about restriction; it's about intention and balance.
You're on vacation. Eat the gelato. Just drink your water, take your walk, and remember: glowing is about balance.

Hotel Room Glow-Up Workouts
You don't need a gym. You need your body and five feet of space.
Travel Reset Workout (10–15 mins):
- 20 air squats

- 10 incline pushups (use the bed or desk)
- 30-second wall sit
- 20 walking lunges
- 15-second plank hold
- Repeat 2x while watching your favorite show
- Bonus move: hold a soup can in each hand and do 15 shoulder presses

Not into circuits? Go for a 15-minute walk around the block or beach and count it.

Reminder: Movement resets mood. No guilt. Just glow.

The Glow Girl Travel Packing List

Skincare + Wellness:

- Zinc sunscreen
- Hydrating mist
- Magnesium spray
- Silk eye mask
- Essential oils
- Organic coconut oil
- Non-LED red light device *see tips

Beauty Tools:

- Hair stick (for that ponytail lift!)
- Clean mascara

- Tinted zinc SPF or BB cream

Food & Drink:

- Seed-oil-free snacks
- Electrolyte packets
- Reusable water bottle
- Tea bags (ginger, mint, or chamomile)

Outfits:

- 2 casual daytime outfits
- 1 dinner-ready outfit
- 1 "I need to feel hot today," look
- 1 comfy lounge set

Now multiply this by 5. Then panic-pack a backup outfit you'll never wear.

Tips + Tricks:

- Why no LED red light? Many LED devices emit blue-spectrum light that disrupts your circadian rhythm and can damage skin. Look for near-infrared, non-LED options that promote collagen and cellular repair.
- Coconut oil? Make it organic—always. It's your moisturizer, hair mask, makeup remover, and snack in one.

- Chlorophyll drops? Only use reputable, clean brands with no synthetic additives.

Weekly Affirmation

"I travel light, glow hard, and make every stop count. I'm 80% clean, 20% carefree, and 100% glowing—snacks packed, cheekbones lifted, and zero guilt in my carry-on."

Chapter 16: Hoarder? No. Archivist of Questionable Fashion Choices

If You Only Buy It Once

You don't need a million outfits. You need a few that make you feel unstoppable.

Your Closet Should Hype You Up, Not Stress You Out

You've been there. The closet's packed, but nothing feels right. Instagram hauls make you feel like you need an entire new wardrobe every season—one minute it's butter yellow cardigans, the next it's ballet-core, then mob-wife fur. But real style? It's not a trend. It's a feeling.

Let's build a wardrobe that works harder than your group chat—elevated, timeless, and unapologetically you.

The Capsule Closet That Glows Year-Round

Top Staples:

- A tailored white tank (thick straps, quality fabric, not see-through)
- A crisp Oxford shirt in white or pale blue (perfect for layering)
- A soft, neutral cashmere or organic cotton sweater
- A structured tee (not your ex's oversized one)

Bottom Essentials:

- High-waisted straight-leg denim (dark wash or bone white)
- Flattering black trousers or tailored wide-legs
- A flowy midi skirt that twirls just right

Outerwear Icons:

- A sharp blazer (go monochrome or camel)
- A classic trench coat (water-resistant but chic)
- A structured cropped jacket or utility layer

Dresses to Rotate:

- A silk slip or matte jersey midi that works day-to-night
- A breezy linen shirt dress (belted if you like)

Shoes That Stick:

- A pair of white leather tennis shoes (not gym shoes)
- Nude or black low block heels
- Minimalist leather sandals
- A walkable boot in a versatile tone

Accessories That Finish the Look:

- Oversized sunglasses (Jackie O always wins)
- Gold hoops or a signature earring
- A sleek neutral crossbody or top-handle tote
- Claw clip or hair stick pomade for that polished ponytail lift

Fabric Matters: Why We Avoid the Plastic Closet

Fast fashion is fun—until it melts in the dryer or clings to you in all the wrong places. Synthetic fabrics like polyester, acrylic, and nylon are literally plastic. They trap sweat, shed microplastics, and mess with your glow (hello, skin irritation). Linen, cotton, and organic blends allow your skin to breathe, regulate temperature, and last for years when properly cared for. Pro tip? That lived-in linen look is effortlessly elegant and only gets better with time.

Look for "100% linen" or "organic cotton" on the label—and skip anything that feels like a shower curtain.

Closet Glow-Up Tips

- Get all one hanger color. You'll feel *lux*—trust me.
- If you haven't worn it in a year, reverse hang it. Still untouched after a season? Donate.
- Build around neutrals you love—black, bone, navy, olive, cream. Then layer in color or print.
- You don't need more. You need better.

Where to Shop (Curated, Not Compulsive)

Forget fast fashion FOMO. You're building your archive.

- Amazon finds (search: organic linen pants, neutral cotton tanks)
- Right now - *Loving H&M's Conscious Collection*
- Local boutiques or eco-conscious brands that list real materials
- Vintage or resale shops *only* if they carry high-quality items—skip the chaos bins

---

Closet Confidence Tracker

Wardrobe Check-In	✓ Completed
Decluttered one category (tops, pants, etc.)	
Replaced plastic hangers with matching ones	
Donated items not worn in a year	
Built one complete outfit from capsule items	
Identified your three go-to colors	
Ordered a quality organic cotton or linen staple	
Reorganized accessories	
Tossed any item made of 100% polyester	
Created a "maybe" pile for a second pass	

Weekly Affirmation:

"I dress like someone worth meeting—because I am. And I refuse to let polyester steal my shine."

Chapter 17: Glow Mode: Chaos + Hacks = Results

Be: Glow shouldn't be high maintenance but a high reward.

Welcome to the ultimate cheat sheet. You've got things to do, places to be, and a tiny window between errands and espresso. These glow hacks are for the days when your ponytail is on hour six, your concealer is creased, and you need something extra without a complete routine reset. These are your Glow Mode SOS moments. Bookmark, screenshot, and share, don't gatekeep them.

Under-Boob Sweat, Be Gone

Arrowroot powder is your best friend. Dust it on like a goddess before a walk, workout, or running errands in the summer heat. Bonus: it's talc-free and toxin-free. Apply with a puff, your hands, or a powder brush.

Make Your Tan Look Expensive (Even if it's DIY)

Use an exfoliating mitt *before* you apply self-tanner. You want smooth skin, not patchy elbows. Moisturize dry spots like ankles and wrists first. Let the product dry fully, and avoid wearing the white tank top for at least an hour. Look for tanners with organic ingredients and skip the synthetic fragrance.

Dry Brush = Instant Lymph Drain + Baby Soft Skin

Before you shower, use a dry brush in upward strokes toward your heart. Start with your feet and work your way up. This exercise stimulates lymph flow, exfoliates dead skin, and helps your body detox naturally. Don't press too hard—unlike sandpaper, it should feel invigorating.

Baking Soda Teeth Polish

Want a brighter smile without bleach? Mix *aluminum-free* baking soda with organic coconut oil and gently brush for a minute. Do it once a week—don't overdo it. You'll get that polished look without the scary dental bills.

Beauty Blender Detox

If you're not careful, your makeup sponge will become a bacteria sponge. Skip the microwave method (seriously, don't)—instead, boil water, pour it into a bowl, and add a few drops of clean castile soap or apple cider vinegar. Let it soak, rinse thoroughly, and air dry in sunlight.

Oil Slick Hair Hack

If your roots are out of control and you don't have dry shampoo, arrowroot powder or organic cornstarch works in a pinch. Just apply a little with a fluffy makeup brush. Start small—you want fresh, not ghostly.

Slicked Ponytail Cheat Code

Flyaways be gone. Use a hair stick (aka hair paste in a twist-up tube) to get that snatched, clean look. The ponytail lift is real—bonus points for a middle part and gold hoops.

Sunglasses = Instant Chic.

Some say too much time in sunglasses can confuse your natural light receptors and disrupt your circadian rhythm, especially in the morning when your body needs natural light to regulate hormones and energy. But we say: rock them *for the pic* and to avoid the sunny squints—big lenses. Bold shapes. Jackie O energy all day long—just be mindful not to block out the sun 24/7. A few minutes of early morning light without shades? That's your real glow starter.

Straw Hack: Because Hydration > Lipstick

Suppose you don't want to mess up your makeup or sip something green that will stain, use a glass or stainless steel straw. Keep one in your bag at all times. It's chic *and* clean.

The Aluminum Swipe Test

Deodorant should not double as a toxin delivery system. Read the label. Aluminum, fragrance, and parabens? Pass. Try magnesium-based or baking soda-free natural sticks. The cleaner your pits, the less you'll notice the transition.

Quick Fix for Puffy Eyes

Two words: frozen spoons. Or a jade roller kept in the fridge. Press gently under your eyes, sip water with electrolytes, and keep blinking—it boosts circulation and makes you look way more awake than you feel.

Glow Mode Mini Challenge: SOS Style

Try three of these hacks this week—just three. Screenshot the list, check them off, and save your favorites for your next panic moment. Glow mode doesn't mean perfect. It means prepared.

Hack	Tried It	Keeping It?
Dry brush before shower	✓	👍 / 👎
Clean up your makeup sponge.	✓	👍 / 👎
Arrowroot powder for sweat	✓	👍 / 👎
Coconut oil + baking soda polish	✓	👍 / 👎
Hair stick ponytail lift	✓	👍 / 👎

Weekly Affirmation

"I don't panic—I pivot. Dry shampoo, under-eye patches, and a little retail therapy never hurt."

Chapter 18: "We've All Googled It"

Stretch marks, loose skin, cellulite—we're talking about all of it. No shame. Just glow.

We've *all* had that late-night Google spiral:

"Why do I look pregnant when I only ate a sandwich?"

"How long until my skin bounces back... asking for a friend (me)?"

"Do stretch marks ever go away, or should I name them?"

"Can you reverse aging with ice rollers and delusion?"

"Does the Target dressing room use funhouse mirrors?"

If you've ever cleared your search history, just in case someone finds it—same. You're in the right place.

And the results? A scroll-hole of ads, before-and-after photos, and $98 miracle serums that leave you confused and discouraged.

Let's cut through it—no shame, no filters—just real solutions for real bodies.

Because It's Not Vanity—It's Self Care

Women of all ages—and whether or not you've been pregnant—worry about things like stretch marks, C-section bumps, cellulite, loose skin, varicose veins, uneven tone, dryness, and puffiness. You're not alone: surveys show around

77% of women report cellulite, uneven tone, dryness, and stretch marks as their top skin concerns.[1]

Here's your compassionate guide to addressing these issues naturally, with research-backed tips and self-love built in.

First, the Glow Mindset

You're not broken. Loose skin, stretch marks, cellulite, hip dips, C-section shelves—whatever's on your list—are normal. Your skin tells a story. But if there's something you want to improve, we support that too. You can love your body and still want to support it. That's not vanity. That's self-respect.

Stretch Marks (Old and New)

The trick here is supporting elasticity and healing from both inside and out.

- Centella Asiatica + hyaluronic acid: A study found that a topical cream with both reduced the appearance of stretch marks by increasing collagen and elastin.

  DIY Tip: Massage organic coconut oil post-shower, then apply a Centella-infused serum or cream.

---

[1] The Benchmarking Company. "2022 PinkReport: Women's Wellness & Personal Care." Accessed June 23, 2025.
https://benchmarkingcompany.com/research/2022-pinkreport-wellness/.

- Organic Rosehip Oil: High in vitamins A and C, this helps fade scars and improve skin tone.

- Micro-needling roller (DIY version): Gently stimulates collagen. Use with a clean tool once a week after applying rosehip oil.

- Hydration: Your skin is an organ—treat it like one. Use filtered water and add a pinch of sea salt or an electrolyte mix without sugar or synthetic dyes.

Loose Skin (Especially Post-Baby or Weight Loss)

This one takes time, but consistency helps.

- Organic Castor Oil Packs: When used 2–3 times a week, these packs support lymphatic drainage and skin firmness. They are messy but worth it.

- Red Light Therapy (non-LED): This naturally stimulates collagen and helps reduce crepey texture. Avoid cheap LED masks. Look for non-LED red light panels or wands, and use caution with your eyes.

- Protein & Collagen: You need the building blocks. Prioritize collagen-rich foods like bone broth or high-quality collagen peptides.

C-Section Shelf / Lower Belly Bump

You're not imagining it. The scar tissue and fascia tension can create that "shelf."

- Massage and Fascia Tools: Help break up adhesions and improve circulation.
- Abdominal Wrapping (Gentle): Not waist trainers! A light, breathable wrap postpartum can help retrain core connection.
- Breathwork and Pelvic Floor Exercises: These are more powerful than crunches. Try the "core canister" breathing method.
- Ab Strength Workouts: Think pelvic tilts, small crunches, and controlled breathing to help tighten skin.
- Dry Brushing Boosts circulation and lymphatic flow.

Be patient—almost every woman is on a journey here.

Cellulite and Skin Texture

- Cellulite is common—90% of women have it.[2] It's about connective tissue, circulation, and inflammation.
- Organic Coffee Scrub with Cinnamon or Ginger: Stimulates circulation and exfoliates. Use 2–3 times a week.
- Dry Brushing (Daily): Always brush toward your heart—start at the feet and work upward before showering.

Skin Discoloration / Uneven Tone

- Azelaic Acid: Naturally brightens and reduces inflammation without bleaching skin. Look for a clean brand with minimal fillers.
- Chlorophyll Drops: Detoxifies and oxygenates skin. Make sure it's from a clean, synthetic-free source.
- Zinc-Based SPF: Choose a non-toxic, mineral-based sunscreen for daily use.

---

[2] Cleveland Clinic. "Cellulite: Causes, Treatments, and Facts." Last reviewed March 8, 2023. https://my.clevelandclinic.org/health/diseases/15572-cellulite.

- Gentle Exfoliation: Sugar scrubs, lactic acid, or enzyme masks help with tone and texture.
- Moisture Layering: Use hyaluronic acid and whipped tallow post-shower for deep hydration.
- Under-eye puffiness: Try a cold jade roller or frozen spoons, hydrate well, and prioritize sleep.

Varicose Veins & Leg Fatigue

About 23% of adults have visible veins.

- Movement: Do calf raises or walk 10 minutes daily.
- Compression Socks: Support blood flow and reduce swelling.
- Add Flavonoid-Rich Foods: Berries, citrus, and leafy greens help strengthen capillaries.
- Horse Chestnut Cream: Supports blood flow and capillary tone.
  Note: Avoid if you have a tree nut allergy or sensitive skin. Always patch test first—glowing legs, not itching ones!

Let's Not Forget the Basics

- Hydrate with electrolytes, not just plain water

- Ditch the seed oils — they inflame everything
- Move daily — even a short walk counts
- Laugh often — joy helps circulation, too

Bonus Basics 101: Vitamin D Deserves a Glow-Up

We said glow starts from within, and that includes the sunshine vitamin. Vitamin D is crucial for hormone balance, bone strength, immune support, and mood stability. But if you're indoors all day or slathered in SPF (which you *should* be—as long as it's chemical-free zinc-based), you might be low.

Ask your doctor to run labs, and if you need a supplement, choose a clean vitamin D3 + K2 blend for better absorption.

Collagen & Peptides: Your Skin's Best Friends

Collagen is the scaffolding that keeps your skin plump, your joints cushioned, and your glow from going ghost. After age 25, production starts to decline (rude, right?).

Add hydrolyzed, grass-fed collagen peptides to your routine. Unflavored powders blend easily into coffee or smoothies. Pair them with vitamin C to help your body use them. I love the ancient nutrition brand supplements for collagen!

Magnesium: Not All Forms Are Created Equal

Magnesium is among the most essential (and underrated) minerals in your glow-up toolkit. It supports stress, sleep, hormones, and digestion, and most women are deficient in it. But before you grab a bottle off the shelf, know this: the form matters. Here's your cheat sheet:

- Magnesium Glycinate → Calms anxiety, supports sleep, helps relax muscles
- Magnesium Citrate → Aids constipation (but can work *too* well—use with caution)
- Magnesium Malate → Boosts energy and muscle function
- Magnesium Threonate → Supports focus and mood (crosses the blood-brain barrier)
- Magnesium Chloride → Found in topical sprays and bath soaks—great for sore muscles
- Magnesium Oxide → Cheap, poorly absorbed, and best skipped

Choose clean brands—no artificial dyes, mystery binders, or synthetic fillers. Look for third-party tested options, ideally paired with vitamin B6 or taurine for optimal absorption.

Think of magnesium like skincare for your insides.
Personalized. Targeted. And glow-inducing.

On My Radar: Colostrum

Okay, hear me out. Yes, it's literally the first milk mammals produce. But colostrum is now being bottled as the *it-girl* of gut health—loaded with growth factors, immune support, and skin-glow potential.

Some swear by it for calming inflammation, healing the gut lining, and even boosting workout recovery. *Still doing my homework, but if you see it on your For You page? You're not alone.*

Weekly Affirmation

"My skin tells a story—but I decide the ending. I glow with grace, not guilt."

Chapter 19: Fine, I'll Glow Then

You made it.

Not just to the end of a book, but through 18 chapters of seed oil slander, closet purges, and probably a few "Wait... is that me?" moments. If you're still reading, I hope you've laughed, learned, taken a screenshot, and maybe even thrown out a bottle of canola oil in rage.

So, where do you go from here?

You don't start over on Monday. You don't wait until the kids are older, your schedule clears, or Mercury directs. You pick one thing. One swap. One habit. And you let it stack.

You glow anyway.

And yes, you actually can do this. Even if your fridge is a mess, your inbox has 3,742 unread emails, and your idea of self-care today was locking the bathroom door with a piece of chocolate. This isn't about perfection—it's about momentum. One better choice. One label read. One supplement that doesn't taste like chalk. You're not behind—you're just not broadcasting your glow-up every five minutes, which makes it even more powerful. This wasn't a manual. It was a glow-up group chat in book form. The kind you open during errands, scroll before bed, or shove at your best friend with a "Read this, it's literally us."

Because let's be honest: you don't need a guru. You need a girl who's been there. Who's Googled: "Is stress making my face weird?" "Can magnesium fix my personality?" and "Best dry shampoo to fake a full life."

And that's me. Hi. It's me.

I didn't write this because I had everything all figured out. I did so after a busy week filled with campaign events, school drop-offs, and quick meals in parking lots—yet people kept asking me about my skincare routine. That's when it hit me: maybe the glow wasn't just luck. Perhaps it's time to share my little secret.

You want answers. And glow. And sleep. But mostly glow.

This book is the sum of what worked and what didn't. It's the "I tried it so you don't have to." It's a hug and a hype session, minus the toxic positivity. It's the vitamin D you didn't know you were missing.

So here's your final reminder: You can glow in the chaos. To shine even if your house looks like a Target clearance aisle and your group chat is 187 messages deep about someone's in-laws and a vacation house full of roaches.

Thank you for trusting me and letting me be in your brain while you folded laundry or panic-Googled "non-toxic sunscreen for toddlers." Thank you for being the woman who wants to learn, laugh, and question the status quo—and do it in lip gloss.

You've got this. You *are* this.

Now make the group chat proud.

With love and a caffeine-fueled vendetta against seed oils,

Margot

P.S. Just in case you forgot what you pulled off:

You didn't just read a book.

You detoxed your beauty bag, broke up with sunflower oil, learned to decode "natural" labels, and figured out why your mascara might be gaslighting you.

You found real-deal grocery swaps, kicked fake wellness out of your cart, and picked up a few things your great-grandmother would actually recognize as food.

You started reading ingredient labels like love letters—and swiping left on the toxic ones.

You purged your closet, flirted with linen, and gave your leggings a sabbatical (unless they're doing their job, in which case: carry on).

You started showing up differently. More aware. More

magnetic. More you.

You learned how to glow on your own terms.

You don't need a before-and-after photo. This whole book was the after.

Now take a screenshot.

Text your best friend.

And start Chapter You.

glow glossary

A cheeky cheat sheet for the casually confused

GLOW MODE – THAT FEELING WHEN YOUR SKIN'S CLEAR, YOUR ERRANDS ARE ROMANTICIZED, AND YOUR FRIDGE HAS GRASS-FED BUTTER.

SEED OIL SLAY – A SARCASTIC TERM FOR WHAT WE'RE NOT DOING. TRANSLATION: AVOIDING INFLAMMATORY OILS LIKE IT'S OUR JOB.

HOT GIRL WALK – A LONG, DRAMATIC WALK WITH SUNGLASSES AND EXISTENTIAL CLARITY.

TALLOWCORE – WHEN YOU REALIZE BEEF FAT WORKS BETTER THAN YOUR $80 CREAM.

MAIN CHARACTER ENERGY – YOU, AFTER 8 HOURS OF SLEEP AND ONE BOUNDARY ENFORCED.

CHAOS + HACKS = RESULTS – OUR FORMULA. UNHINGED BUT GLOWING.

COPY-PASTE INFLUENCERS – THE GIRLS WHO ALL LOOK THE SAME AND RECOMMEND ALMOND MILK WITH 15 INGREDIENTS. NOT OUR VIBE.

THE GROUP CHAT – YOUR REAL FRIENDS. OR THIS BOOK. OR BOTH.

INGREDIENT DETECTIVE – THE GIRL AT THE GROCERY ZOOMING IN ON LABELS LIKE SHE'S DECODING A CIA FILE. SPOILER: IT'S YOU NOW.

ERRANDS, BUT MAKE IT PRETTY – WHETHER IT'S SCHOOL DROP-OFF, GROCERY RUNS, OR JUST PRETENDING TO HAVE ERRANDS SO YOU CAN VIBE IN YOUR CAR, YOU ROLLED UP IN TINTED SPF AND LIP OIL. YOU'RE NOT JUST GOING— YOU'RE GLOWING.

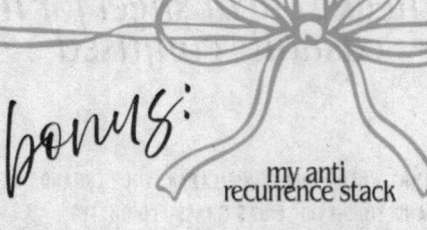

my anti recurrence stack

Let's keep it real: this is not a shopping list. I don't expect you to buy out an entire wellness aisle. But I do want to be transparent. This is the exact protocol I follow to support healing and reduce my risk of cancer recurrence. It's what I researched, vetted, and refined over time—always choosing non-synthetic, clean options. This is not medical advice. It's what I do based on my health history, and I worked with my doctor. Please consult yours, check your levels, and remember —real food > pills. But this stack pulls its weight when life gets busy or you need support. As mentioned in the manuscript, I use Ancient Nutrition collagen in smoothies or coffee! Think of this as a peek inside my cabinet:

ASTAXANTHIN
SUPPORTS SKIN ELASTICITY, PROTECTS AGAINST UV AND BLUE LIGHT, AND REDUCES OXIDATIVE STRESS.
FOOD TWIN: WILD SALMON, SHRIMP, RED MICRO ALGAE
FAV BRAND: BIOASTIN

NAC + MILK THISTLE
BOOSTS GLUTATHIONE (YOUR MASTER DETOXIFIER), SUPPORTS IMMUNITY AND CELLULAR REPAIR.
FOOD TWIN: COOKED SPINACH, ASPARAGUS, GARLIC, AND ARTICHOKES
FAV BRAND: MERCOLA

VITAMIN D3 + K2 , ZINC & SELENIUM
STRENGTHENS IMMUNE FUNCTION AND HELPS REGULATE ABNORMAL CELL GROWTH. ZINC SUPPORTS SKIN HEALING AND HORMONE BALANCE; SELENIUM HELPS YOUR BODY NEUTRALIZE OXIDATIVE STRESS AND SUPPORTS THYROID FUNCTION.
FOOD TWIN: PASTURED EGG YOLKS, SARDINES, GRASS-FED BUTTER, BRAZIL NUTS, OYSTERS, PUMPKIN SEEDS, AND EGGS
FAV BRAND: PURE ENCAPSULATION

CURCUMIN
A POWERFUL ANTI-INFLAMMATORY AND ANTI-CANCER COMPOUND THAT HELPS REGULATE CELL HEALTH.
FOOD TWIN: TURMERIC ROOT (WITH BLACK PEPPER)
FAV BRAND: ORGANIC INDIA TURMERIC

MEDICINAL MUSHROOMS
REISHI AND TURKEY TAIL SUPPORT IMMUNE RECOGNITION AND RESPONSE TO ABNORMAL CELLS.
FOOD TWIN: TOUGH TO GET IN EVERYDAY FOODS UNLESS YOU'RE A FORAGER
FAV BRAND: REAL MUSHROOMS

OMEGA-3S (KRILL OIL)
REDUCES INFLAMMATION, SUPPORTS SKIN HEALING, AND PROTECTS AGAINST CELL MUTATIONS.
FOOD TWIN: MACKEREL, SARDINES, ANCHOVIES, WILD SALMON
FAV BRAND: MERCOLA

LIPOSOMAL GLUTATHIONE
SUPPORTS DETOX, ESPECIALLY DURING STRESS, TOXIN EXPOSURE, OR RECOVERY.
FAV BRAND: PURE ENCAPSULATION

SHILAJIT RESIN
A MINERAL-DENSE ADAPTOGEN THAT SUPPORTS MITOCHONDRIA, HORMONE BALANCE, AND CLEAN ENERGY.
FAV BRAND: CYMBIOTIKA OR PURE HIMALAYAN

About The Author

She's read the studies. She's tested the hacks. She's probably in your group chat.

Margot Reed might not be real, but her glow is.
She's the girl you *think* you saw in Pilates last week, the one in the high-tight pony and chocolate Relyte-stained travel mug. She's read all the wellness blogs, so you don't have to, and she's probably already ordered the thing you're about to Google.

Is she a nutritionist? No. A dermatologist? Also no.
She's dangerously good at reading ingredient labels and discovering what "invisible inflammation" means, ensuring you're always one step ahead in your wellness journey.

She's that elusive friend who knows the exact sunscreen to wear to brunch and the one supplement that made a difference.

Margot Reed writes under a pen name because she once signed an NDA so intense, it practically came with its own legal team.

She's part internet myth, part accidental BFF, always ready to share a wellness tip or two.
Some say she's a former beauty editor with a skincare fridge full of secrets. Others swear she's under NDA from a wellness brand so big it can't be named. The truth? She's the anonymous bestie behind *Holy Glow Grail*, here to spill the tea on seed oils, toxic products, and why your face might be mad at your moisturizer.

Margot doesn't have a blue check. She has something better: a brain full of research, a bathroom full of tallow, and an adult life built on unique wellness practices. She's not about filters, gatekeeping, or wellness cults—just one glow-hacked chapter at a time.

She might reveal her real name someday. Until then, the mystery of Margot Reed continues...
XOXO,
You-Know-Who

P.S.
This book may be over, but the glow-up isn't.
Join the email—it's like a clean girl cult minus the weird robes.
Scan below!

If this book made you laugh, learn, or dramatically side-eye your pantry... leave a glowing Amazon review. Drop your favorite line in the review—yes, the one you screenshotted for the group chat. Text your besties, share the glow. I'm reading every word (probably with an iced coffee in hand), and yes, your glow energy is noticed! And for the tips too juicy to print, follow on Instagram: @holyglowgrail

Your Glow Goals and Random Thoughts

Your Glow Goals and Random Thoughts

Your Glow Goals and Random Thoughts